THE TRUTH ABOUT A VEGETARIAN DIET

The Research that made one Meat Eater Go Green -
*Dispelling the biggest myths of being a
Vegetarian*

Clay Elston

COMPLIMENTARY BONUSES

To make sure you get the most value out of this book, here are three exclusive resources that will help you on your "plant-based" journey.

1. 1000 Vegetarian Recipes

We compiled 1000 delicious recipes for all occasions and it is yours for purchasing this book on Amazon. You'll never need another recipe book again!

2. Juice Cheat Sheet

This is a one page print off with 24 of my favourite juices. Print it off and stick it in your kitchen. It's the perfect "cheat sheet" when you need to get your 'juices' flowing!

3. All Time Favourite Recipes

This is a beautifully designed curated collection of our favourite recipes.

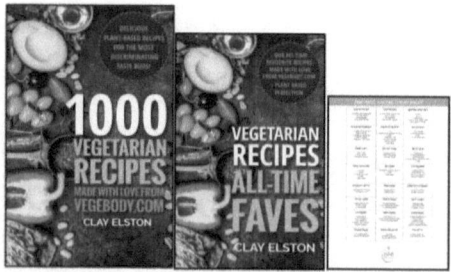

You can download these resources here:
www.vegebody.com/amazongifts

Any questions, please don't hesitate to contact me at www.vegebody.com.

<u>DISCLAIMER</u>

The Truth about a Vegetarian Diet

Clay Elston

All rights reserved.

Copyright ©2016 by Clay Elston.

Many hours from many helpers (proof-readers, editors, designers, friends, kindle book formatters) has gone into making this little book a resource that provides value to you, the reader. The aim is to deliver value to the reader and is designed for you and I hope you like it enough to leave a five-star review (although, any review at all would be lovely to receive!).

Special thanks to all who helped contribute directly and indirectly to the publication of this book. Enjoy.

<u>WHO AM I?</u>

My name is Clay and I have been "plant-strong" for over a decade. I have a couple of plant-based digital businesses and am a member of numerous vegetarian organisations in the Australasia community. In addition to being "plant-based", I'm also an avid traveller and fitness enthusiast. My home is based in beautiful Sydney, Australia.

The purpose of this book is to provide a research-backed perspective on the benefits of being vegetarian... without the fluff. There has been far too few books written on this subject and I hope I can do this topic justice. I hope you find value within these pages and are then able to "vegucate" others on plant-based eating.

If you have any questions about going "plant strong", let me know at www.vegebody.com.

Until then, enjoy!
Much gratitude,

Clay Elston

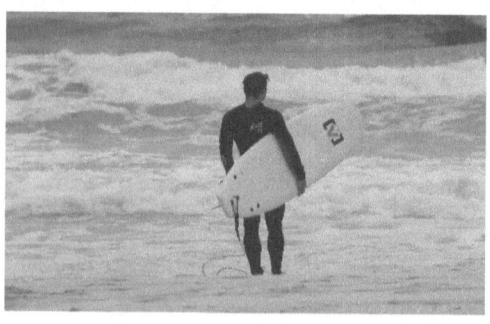

CONTENTS

Complimentary Bonuses.................................... 2

Disclaimer.. 3

Who Am I?.. 4

Chapter One: Introduction 6

Chapter Two: Where Do You Get Your Protein? 8

Chapter Three: Don't You Need Meat To Grow?........ 15

Chapter Four: What Can You Eat?........................ 22

Chapter Five: Where Do You Get Your Calcium, Iron,

    And Omega-3s?....................................... 25

Chapter Six: What's Good About A Vegetarian Diet,

    Anyway? 31

Chapter Seven: Isn't It Difficult Going Vegetarian?.... 35

Chapter Eight: How Can An Elite Athlete Be

    Plant-Based?.. 39

Chapter Nine: Conclusion.............................. 45

Recommended Resources 46

Don't Forget Your Complimentary

Bonuses! 48

Thanks For Reading. Now, What?.................... 49

CHAPTER ONE: INTRODUCTION

This book has taken me a few years to finally start writing. I'd like to say what got me started was divine intervention, a new productivity-hack or an amazing super-green smoothie, but it's a lot simpler than that. I simply ran out of reasons (read "excuses') for why I don't have the authority to write this book. After all, there are many more individuals in this industry with more authority, talent, and credibility and although they didn't directly contribute to writing this book, they have all helped play a part in the creation of the information in it. Standing on the shoulders of these gentle giants is, after all, what research is all about! I hope this short book helps shed some light on why you should consider becoming "plant-based", if you haven't already.

First of all, thank you for reading this book. If you have any questions at all please do not hesitate to contact me when you're finished. My team and I have also done our best to make sure we have crammed in as much value for your dollars as we could (which, thanks to Kindle, is less than the price of a Starbucks coffee!). Each myth is kept sweet and simple, as you have enough on your metaphorical "plate."

To be clear, the intention of a plant-based diet isn't just about giving up meat. It's actually about gaining. It's about vitality. It's about running on a more efficient fuel source. It's about optimal living. But at the same time, it's really about building towards better health. Pure and simple.

You will not find any negative preaching here. Besides... we're optimists. With the amount of positive research-backed studies conducted in the last decade, getting your "V-Plates" is easier than ever before.

Even with many compelling studies on plant-based eating, we have over a century of conditioning that has created many stereotypes and myths that are deeply engrained in most of us and need busting. Here we cover some of the biggest "myth-busting" questions such as;

1. **Where do you get your protein?**
2. **Don't you need meat to grow?**
3. **What can you eat?**
4. **Where do you get your calcium, iron, and omega-3's?**
5. **What's so great about a vegetarian diet?**
6. **Isn't it difficult going vegetarian?**
7. **How can an elite athlete eat plant-based?**

Stay tuned for the next chapter when we'll get into the question, where do vegetarians really get their protein? We've tackled this from all angles, so hopefully you'll find it a good read.

CHAPTER TWO: WHERE DO YOU GET YOUR PROTEIN?

"Whenever you find yourself on the side of the majority, it is time to pause and reflect."
- Mark Twain

So, where do you get your protein?!

Personally, I definitely don't look like I am missing "protein" nor do most vegetarians, but the urge for many individuals when meeting a vegetarian is to instantly become a novice nutritionist or dietician.

If you have been plant-based for a while, you will have inevitably come across somebody, somewhere, asking you this question. Mention that you are one of those "V" words and the conversation starts going down the rabbit hole.

My answer usually depends upon the sincerity behind the deeper meaning of the question.

Without getting too deep, it shows society's belief that meat is synonymous with protein! Thanks to multimillion-dollar marketing media blitz starting in the 50's, our culture unknowingly turned us into "walking billboards" for the meat and dairy industry. The average person's understanding of protein is that it is derived solely from meat and dairy. A more fascinating question is finding out the truth of making the switch.

I've split this chapter into three sections.

Section one will answer "What is protein?" Section two will look at some interesting stuff you ought to know about protein, and section three will look at the sources of plant-based protein.

By the time you finish this chapter, you'll be among the minority of people who actually know what they're talking about when it comes to protein.

What is Protein?

When people ask, "How much protein should I eat?" what they are really asking is, "Which amino acids does my body need, in which quantity do I need them and to what degree are the foods containing them digestible and not disruptive to my personal metabolism when ingested?" Complicated? Sure, but let me explain…

There are only a few "essential" things you need to know about protein.

Protein is the basic machinery of all your cells (and those cells make up your *entire* body). Proteins are made up of acids called amino acids. Amino acids are the *real* "building blocks" and are crucial for maintaining and regulating your body. There are only 21 amino acids that your body needs. Most of these your body can synthesize itself, but nine of them it cannot. These nine must come from your food intake. These nine amino acids are called ‚essential amino acids' because it is essential that you get them through your food! If you are lacking even one, your body is out of balance. There are few types of foods that contain all the essential amino acids, which is why we need to eat a variety of foods.

Unlike your favourite mix-and-match outfits, amino acids are not interchangeable and can't be stored for later use. Therefore, we must ingest each amino acid roughly in the proportion we require it every day. Our biological needs are for specific amino acids in specific proportions, but "protein" can mean *any combination of one or more amino acids.* Therefore, the amount of "protein" in food is, by itself, a nearly meaningless number.

Things You Should Know About Protein

There is far too much emphasis on protein.

Most people have no idea what the ideal amount of protein is. We have been conditioned to think that protein is provided by just meat and dairy foods. If you know someone who thinks like this, read the latest study on protein absorption, linked in your resource section of this book.

Many well-known plant-based proponents (such as Dr. McDougal, Dr. Colin Campbell, Caldwell Esselstyn MD) support the notion that you actually need very little protein. Let's look at a basic example: gorillas and bananas. Bananas are 1-4% protein. Does a 100-pound gorilla look like it is lacking protein?

We are obviously not gorillas, although genetically we share 98% of our DNA with gorillas. The current recommended daily allowance for protein for the average adult is 0.8-1.0 milligrams/kilogram body weight. This includes a safe margin of error. For most people, a sufficient protein intake will be 10-20% of their daily calories. Athletes in training or those recovering from illness need more. It is also interesting to note that the RDA of protein has doubled since the 1970s. A controversial point argued here is that many activists believe this was due to behind-the-scenes lobbying from the dairy industry.

Let's look at the question another way. Have you ever heard of anyone suffering from a protein deficiency?! A blue moon is more common than protein deficiencies in the developed world. Problems arising from too much protein, however, are far more common.

An important consideration to remember about protein is that by calorie intake, many green vegetables have more protein than meat. Broccoli, for instance, has 11.1 grams per calories of protein, whereas a porterhouse steak has only 6.5 grams. Of course, a lot more broccoli is needed (about two cups) to reach the same caloric intake. Broccoli also comes packed with a bevy of vitamins, calcium, and cancer-preventing qualities. There is more contention over this issue than what it's worth, but the biggest takeaway is that there is more protein in vegetables than most realize.

The science around the importance of protein is not clear, but societies that consume high levels of animal protein do have higher levels of cancer – though whether this is caused by the excess meat or reduced consumption of cancer-fighting foods such as fruits and vegetables is not known. The International Agency for Research on Cancer reports that the regions with the highest incidence of cancer are Australia/New Zealand, Western Europe, and North America, all of which consume high levels of meat and dairy. Those with the lowest incidence of cancer are Eastern Asia, Northern

Africa, and South-Central Asia. Furthermore, the countries that consume low amounts of animal proteins (including dairy foods), such as African and Asian countries also show extremely low rates of osteoporosis.

Meanwhile, in the American Journal of Clinical Nutrition, Dr. Luigi Fontana stated that "many people are eating too many animal products – such as meat, cheese, eggs and butter – as well as refined grains and free sugars." He believes that diets would be healthier if we ate more wholegrains, beans, fruits and vegetables and far fewer animal products.

One last thing about protein that you should know. Timing is everything. This is especially true when it comes to muscle growth. Most people have enough protein at dinner but are lacklustre when it comes to their daytime meals. Protein is vital for many more reasons besides muscle development. A better question to ask yourself is, "When am I getting my protein?" Research by the University of Connecticut found that the muscle building growth of men who ate protein every few hours was significantly higher than it was in those who ate protein at once over a longer time span.

Now let's look at protein sources.

Where do Vegetarians get their Protein?

Everywhere.

There it is! That's your answer! All foods you eat contain protein. If it's a whole food, it has protein.

Legumes, nuts and vegetables are excellent sources of protein. Here are seven of my favourite sources.

1. 1 burrito with rice, beans, and vegetables = 40 grams protein

2. 1 cup tempeh = 30 grams protein

3. 1 cup quinoa = 26 grams protein

4. 1 large salad with vegetables, sunflower seeds, and raisins = 20 grams protein

5. 1 cup tofu = 18 grams protein

6. 1 falafel sandwich with 3 balls, hummus and tahini = 18 grams protein

7. 1 cup cooked lentils = 16 grams protein

To show you how simple it is to reach your body's protein needs, let's take a look at average Pete, who weighs an average 75 kilograms. It is recommended that Pete eats 60-75 grams of protein per day. One cup of tempeh is 30 grams of protein and a burrito with rice, beans and vegetables is 40 grams. That equals 70 grams! Booyah. Wasn't that easy? If you want protein-loaded recipes, you'll find some in the bonus gifts at the beginning and end of this book.

If you find that getting enough protein is hard, try upping your eggs (unless you are vegan) or try a spinach tofu scramble. If you are short on time, there are many awesome plant-based protein supplements. There are now many types, such as rice, soy, almond, pea, quinoa, etc., and I would recommend getting a mixed blend as well as one that you enjoy the taste of. A lot of them mix easier than whey-based protein, and the taste for most is a lot better.

The next time someone asks you where you get your protein, suppress the urge to scream in frustration and take the opportunity to not just educate, but "**veg**ucate". Alternatively, you can be a ‚smarty pants', and answer with "I get it from Tempeh: 24gms, Lentils: 17.9gms, Quinoa: 11gms, Spirulina 68% and of course, nuts". Your choice!

Now let's get into Chapter Three: "Don't you need meat to grow?"

CHAPTER THREE: DON'T YOU NEED MEAT TO GROW?

Here's a bold statement:

Increasing your vegetarian-based food intake will create an improvement in every individual. No exception.

An even bolder statement is that a plant-based diet will promote increased muscle mass and strength. Controversial? For sure! But the devil is in the detail, if you plan on building lean muscles. Sounds like an oxymoron, doesn't it? Thanks to decades of advertising, it does too many people. Let's try and explain, shall we?

Just because you say "no" to meat doesn't mean you have to say "no" to your fitness or muscle building goals.

Let's face it. The stereotype of a vegetarian (and worse, a vegan) isn't doing us any favours. It doesn't exactly conjure up someone who is in peak physical and mental condition oozing with athleticism, does it? Ripped, tanked, shredded or even words like bodybuilding, Olympian or gold medals are not synonymous with going "plant-based"... but maybe they should be.

If you want to make some paradigms shifts, check out our list of famous vegetarian athletes on www.vegebody.com. Former Mr. Universe Bill Pearl and six-time Ms. Olympia Cory Everson are just some of the eye-popping physiques that were both supported by a vegetarian diet.

In the last chapter, we covered what protein really is. But in terms of muscle building, you need to increase your food intake and marginally increase your protein intake.

Muscle building is never just about food. It's much more than that. I use the acronym MESA to help others remember that food is only one part of the puzzle. All are common-sense-based, but you need to remember that at the end of the day all four things need to be in order.

M in MESA stands for MINDSET. Never underestimate the power of the mind in affecting your body.

E is for what you EAT. Eating for any fitness goal is always the most important, but most variable, part.

S is for SLEEP. Rest and sleep help with recovery and muscle replenishing.

A is for ACTIVITY. Whether it is fitness training, running, sports or yoga, the activity is where you put your muscles to the test.

By improving in each category (Mindset, Eat, Sleep, and Activity), you will compound your progress and get phenomenal results. MESA is what it will take to achieve a new level of fitness. Actually, the meaning of the word MESA is an elevated area of land with a flat top and sides that are usually steep cliffs. So expect an initial struggle, but once you are up there, the view is worth it.

Regardless of whether you are a meat-eater or a vegetarian, the principle for building muscle remains the same. You work out anaerobically (i.e. in the gym) and then you consume the necessary nutrients to help your body recover and grow bigger and stronger muscles. Afterwards, you get plenty of "R & R" and keep the right mental attitude. Easy.

The basics of muscle-building workouts haven't changed much over the years. New research and technology have helped us understand the inner workings of particular muscles, and new gym equipment has helped us target specific muscles.

Basic muscle-building exercises should set the foundation for your training regime. This doesn't mean that you are stuck with the same old-school workouts from days of yore. Just stick with their old-school work ethic. Besides, if everyone working out is just following the same training system, there shouldn't be much disparity in their level of fitness, right? But there is, and this is where going plant strong with MESA can make the difference.

There are those who are stronger and faster, and who seem to be more athletically gifted, and this is true for both vegetarians and non-vegetarians. While it's easy to attribute exceptional athletic abilities to genetics, research conducted on the training regime used by both elite vegetarian and non-vegetarian athletes strongly suggests that simple variations in your training, nutritional plans and even rest patterns can bring about vast improvements in your fitness levels and athletic performance.

Effective muscle and strength-building workouts need to be intense, executed with proper form. You don't want your body to adapt to the same workout. Intense, effective training makes the body grow provided that you have a well-balanced and nutrient-filled diet.

For example, those who are working out and looking to put on mass should start with the 40-30-30 macronutrient ratio on a 3,000- to 6,000-calorie-a-day diet (depending on your weight). Don't let the numbers scare you into thinking that it is a huge amount of calories to take in. Remember that you are trying to bulk up, so don't shy away from the very calories your body needs to pack on those muscles.

After you have set goals and know the number of calories you require, think about how you can effectively consume all these calories. Eating large and heavy meals may feel good once in a while, but these are not the kind of meals you want to be eating for health and fitness. It's best to break up the calories into 6-8 small meals throughout the day. Adopt a graze mentality. For this example, we should keep in mind some high-caloric, nutritious food choices that are excellent for bodybuilding and the type of diet we are looking to adopt. Examples of these foods would be nuts/seeds, honey, fruits (especially bananas and coconuts), salads, nut butter, granola, quinoa, potatoes, yams, and avocados. These foods all have a few things in common: they taste great but have a concentrated quota of nutrients, making them dense and highly caloric. Consider eating an orange (60 calories), which delivers a lot of fiber along with vitamin C and juice; however, a glass of orange juice would come from at least 2-3 oranges, amounting to a whopping 180 calories minus the fiber and natural nutrition.

Most vegetarian food choices are naturally low in calories. Because fruits and vegetables are the main constituents and have a high water content, they can make you feel full much faster than non-vegetarian foods. This quality of vegetarian diets is extremely helpful when planning meals. A burst of calories packed in a small fruit or vegetable is the perfect snack while low-calorie vegetarian meals are perfect for nutrition and feeling full. Contrary to popular belief, a balance of calories and nutrition is very easy to handle with a vegetarian menu. Not only that, a few additions and tweaks will easily pack in calories.

If you often feel low on energy and fatigued while training, there is a good chance that your calorie intake is inadequate to support your activity level. When this happens, reevaluate your calorie intake and adjust the calories or workout to complement each other. A lack of calories may make you feel frustrated and want to quit altogether, and we don't want that!

Conversely, the 40-30-30 macronutrient ratio may need to be adjusted for some individuals. This is why you should keep track of your progress. There are a few factors to consider when you are trying to figure out the best macronutrient ratio for yourself. This includes your goals, age, gender, body type, and current fitness level. You know your body best; if you feel that your progress is slow because of the 40-30-30 ratio, try adjusting the distribution by 5%. Be careful not to make drastic changes, as it can throw off your whole training regime.

Finally, while your workouts may tire you out, a good night's rest is imperative for serious training. Sleep rejuvenates the mind and body. It is the best way to recover properly and relieve any slight muscle soreness.

Tips for Building Muscles

1. DRINK TWO PLANT-BASED PROTEIN SHAKES EVERY DAY. Add a scoop of protein and you're in the protein-packing loop. Personally, I'm not a fan of whey powder as it is effectively a byproduct. There are much better sources out there that are closer to nature: rice, almond, hemp, pea and soy protein powders. I would also recommend a higher protein mixed blend content (anywhere from 50-80% is good) as you want to use these after working out and at night.

2. GET A "BULLET," JUICER OR BLENDER. Either way, you'll be downing more healthful nutrients, sending your body into its muscle-building mode. I personally use the Nutri Ninja. It has been the best kitchen tool for me and is often my travelling companion. If you're after some healthy juice recipes, download the complimentary recipes in the bonus kit at the end of this book.

3. EAT BREAKFAST. Get 30 grams of protein into your body within 30 minutes of waking up. It will get your metabolism kick-started and will power up your day. Also, consider "Tofu Tanking" your breakfast. If you don't Tofu, you haven't had the right tofu. If you're not a fan,

try flavoured tofu. Work your way backwards. If you absolutely loathe it, you haven't tried the right tofu!

4. SUPPLEMENT WHEN NECESSARY. If you are unable to get something from food or feel that you are "lacking" a nutrient, don't be afraid to supplement. Consider getting some blood work done next time you are at the doctor to see if you have a nutrient deficiency. Supplements are useful whether you are a vegetarian or not. If you are doing substantial exercise every day, having the right nutrients will help your progress. If you are using workout supplements, go stimulant-free and read the label – not the advertising!

5. COMPOUND EXERCISE AND PROGRESSIVE OVERLOADING. If you are building muscle, you can't go past compound exercises. These are movements that use more than one muscle group at the same time. They are the surest, fastest way to put on quality muscle mass. Add to this an element of progressive overloading, which requires a gradual increase in volume, intensity, frequency or time, to achieve the targeted goal.

CHAPTER FOUR: WHAT CAN YOU EAT?

Even though you are omitting all meat sources, you'll find that you are rewarded many times over with the increase of alternative plant-based sources that you would never have considered. There are a lot of delicious, out-of-the-ordinary plant-based foods that are waiting to be tried. Let's take a look at the many things you should be consuming.

Vegetables and Fruits

This should be obvious. I mean, "vegetarian" and "vegetable" are very nearly the same word (although, the word was derived from "vegetus," meaning lively and vigorous). The longer you stay on the plant-based path, the more you will be exposed (and want to be exposed) to the nutrient filled vegetables. I'm not one for feelings, but you will also start "feeling" the benefits of certain foods and their effects on your body. Asparagus, blueberries, kale, broccoli and bananas are a few of my personal favourites. Bananas make the perfect pre-workout energy boost. Also, there are so many fantastic ways to eat your vegetables and fruits! You can cook, steam, grill, fry, boil, or eat them raw. The fresher you can buy them, the tastier they'll be. You can get a lot of vitamins and minerals and a complete array of amino acids from your vegetables and fruits. They are also the easiest foods for your body to digest!

Beans, Nuts, Legumes, Soy

One of the main things people worry about when they first become vegetarians is how they are going to get enough protein. Any kind of bean or nut is high in protein – some more than others. Soybean is a jack-of-all-trades bean, as it is used in everything. Always opt for an unsweetened soymilk and use it in moderation. Also, as a vegetarian, you will need to get around five servings of beans, nuts, legumes or soy every single day to get enough protein in your diet.

Grains

The word "grains" refers to a multitude of products, including rice, wheat, oats and barley, to name a few. When it comes to ‚supergrains', these are the five you need to eat.

1. Quinoa (pronounced "keen-wah"). This humble grain has the highest nutritional profile of all grains and also comes packed with protein and energy.

2. Amaranth is another high-protein super grain. It contains 50% more protein than most grains. It's been originally grown by the ancient Aztecs over 6000 years ago and now has been part of numerous studies for improving cardiovascular disease and hypertension.

3. Rye is very nutrient-dense and also has low gluten content. It provides a good release of energy.

4. Kamut. What's kamut?! It's a grain that has more protein than an egg. Perfect for us active vegetarians. It's called the "high-energy wheat". It's also one of Dr. Oz's favourites.

5. Buckwheat. This grain is great for your circulation and helps reduce bad cholesterol levels.

A special mention goes to the chia seeds. Although they are theoretically seeds, they have many of the same benefits as grains. They are one of the biggest plant sources of omega-3 fatty acids. Research has also shown that they help reduce diastolic blood pressure. Not bad for just ‚seeds'.

Substitutes

You can find a wide range of substitutes for meat and animal products. If you want a meat-type main course, you can always choose tofu or tempeh. Tofu, treated correctly, may become a "new best friend" and when cooked with a bit of magic, can taste like almost anything you want it to. You can try using tofu in stir-fries, or incorporate it into the main course where meat would usually go. Some people even put tofu in their soups or stews.

If you've decided to give up animal products altogether, there are a wide variety of dairy substitutes available. A few examples include rice, soy, coconut or almond milk and cheese. You can also try a juice bar or make ice cream at home using any of these substitutes.

CHAPTER FIVE: WHERE DO YOU GET YOUR CALCIUM, IRON, AND OMEGA-3s?

The haters will keep on hating the vegetarian diet because, hey, you know, depriving yourself of steaks, that just ain't living! They'll say, "How do you get your nutrients?" "You need meat, eggs and dairy to live, or you'll wither away and die from malnutrition, right?"

Wrong. Dead wrong.

Plant-powered foods are actually the key to getting the right nutrients. Your current mindset may need a bit of tweaking to understand where nutrients come from. With a bit more research and your own self-experimentation, your nutrition knowledge will become not just power, but plant-based power!

The Big C: Calcium

When most people think of calcium, the first type of food that usually comes to mind is dairy. It is a mammoth of a myth that you can get calcium only from cow milk. Kudos goes to the dairy industry as it has even got its own category on the food pyramid. If you are a lacto-ovo vegetarian, you will already be consuming dairy, but for those who want to go without, a change in the "milk" mindset is needed.

A 2009 study by Amy Lanou in The American Journal of Clinical Nutrition shows that although cow milk has been widely recommended in Western countries as necessary for growth and bone health, evidence collected during the past 20 years shows a need to rethink strategies for building and maintaining strong bones. Osteoporotic bone fracture rates are highest in countries that consume the most dairy and animal protein. Most studies of fracture risk provide little or no evidence that milk or other dairy products benefit bone development. Accumulating evidence shows that consuming milk or dairy products may actually contribute to the risk of prostate and ovarian cancers, autoimmune diseases and some childhood ailments. This is obviously a contentious statement; however, it has been supported by various other studies since. Meta-analyses of these studies on milk consumption show fracture risk and osteoporosis have no reduction with high intakes of milk or dairy.

Regardless of your personal opinion, it's becoming clearer to the scientific community that dairy has never been the best source of calcium. So, what are the best sources of calcium? They come from nature. Here's a few to consider:

Kale (1 cup contains 180 milligrams), Blackstrap molasses (2 tablespoons contain 400 milligrams), tempeh (1 cup contains 215 milligrams), turnip greens (1 cup contains 250 milligrams), fortified non-dairy milk (1 cup contains 200-300 milligrams), fortified orange juice (1 cup contains 300 milligrams), figs (1/2 cup contains 120 milligrams) and amaranth (1 cup contains 275 milligrams).

To absorb calcium effectively, the body needs to have an adequate amount of vitamin D. No matter how much calcium you get, it's futile if you aren't getting enough vitamin D, and due to our sedentary lives, that's most of us. Your body synthesizes vitamin D from exposure to sunlight, but if you don't get much sun, you will need to include enough vitamin D in your diet. Eat more mushrooms and eggs. You can also get this vitamin in supplement form or in fortified vegan foods such as soy or rice milk. But the best source is nature. If you have a lunch break today, spend some time in the sun.

'Iron-Up' Your Body with Iron

First of all, if you take your health seriously (and you wouldn't be reading this if you didn't), you need to know why getting enough iron is crucial for your exercise efforts. A lack of iron can seriously affect your mojo, decrease your performance levels and leave you feeling lethargic. In severe cases it leads to anemia.

So, let's get to it; which foods can you count on to give your body enough iron to keep energy pumping through your veins? Some of the best sources include dried fruit, nuts, legumes, spinach, chickpeas, tofu and leafy vegetables (dark green).

Aim for about 15 to 16 milligrams of iron a day, which isn't difficult to achieve. For example, iron-fortified cereals may contain about 18 milligrams per serving, which in itself provides enough iron. Leafy vegetables have about 1 to 3 milligrams of iron per cup, and legumes have almost double that amount per cup. Also, go easy on the caffeine and dairy, as research shows that they impair iron absorption. Instead, consume food or drinks that are rich in vitamin C as this helps the body absorb iron. In other words, forget that extra coffee fix and go for a fruit fix instead!

The Brain Booster: Omega Fats

Chances are you already know that omega-3 is important for your brain, but did you know that this essential Latin lexicon is for your heart, lungs, and immune system? I can't emphasize enough how important getting omega 3, 6 and 9's are for your health. Make sure you get adequate omega fats into your body daily.

You need two servings a day, or about 1000 milligrams, to keep your body adequately nourished with this body booster. Some foods rich in omega-3 fats include chia seeds, flaxseeds and flaxseed oil, hemp seeds, canola, soybean, or walnut oil, tofu, cooked soybeans, hummus, brussel sprouts, sea vegetables and algae. You can also get omega-3 in eggs, which can help fulfill your daily omega-3 quota. Also, if you have been conditioned to think that all this is missing something… well, fishy… you should rethink your thinking.

A Word on Supplementation

I recently attended a health conference where the discussion revolved around supplementation. The conversation revolved around taking multivitamins, and the consensus was if you think it will help, then take them. Like most medicines, the power of the placebo effect comes into account.

Multivitamins have received a bad rap in recent years, with some studies indicating that they provide no benefit or do more harm than good. The backstory for most of these studies is that they were limited in their scope and size. Some of them also had dosages much higher than those in any normal multivitamin.

The first truly sizable and significant study from the National Cancer Institute shows that a daily dose of Centrum Silver multivitamins reduced the total risk of cancer in study participants by 8%. This research included nearly 15,000 male doctors older than 50 for up to 13 years between 1997 and 2011. Before you go out and buy Centrum Silver multivitamins, keep in mind that Dr. J. Michael Gaziano, who conducted the study, only trialled this vitamin because he thought it was a quality product and a brand that would "last the length of his study." It could have been any quality multivitamin which could potentially provide similar results. The point is not to discount multivitamins if you think they will work.

If you are considering taking a multivitamin, make sure it is made by a reputable brand. Also, read the labels and find the brands that have closer to 100% of the daily value of most vitamins and minerals. If you think you are nutrient deficient, see a doctor and get your levels checked. Most people have a magnesium deficiency, however, you won't know if this includes you until you see your results. One general rule is that most vitamins in powder form are better than capsules.

Final thoughts

So, that's calcium, iron, and omega-3s.

As you see, running on ‚plant power' does not leave you with these three most commonly supposed deficiencies. Whatever the nutrients people believe a vegetarian lacks

– whether it is iron, calcium, omega-3, vitamin B12, vitamin D – the deficiency always comes from a lack of understanding. There is no reason why a plant-based person who eats a healthy diet can become deficient in any nutrient. You'll eventually find out that the opposite is true; by eating life-enhancing foods, you'll be nutritionally-efficient. Unfortunately, ,plant-strong platters' are outnumbered, so we are naturally on the defense when it comes to these questions. Eat well and you'll be a living, breathing example to show how strong our ,defense' really is.

CHAPTER SIX: WHAT'S GOOD ABOUT A VEGETARIAN DIET, ANYWAY?

This is a question most often asked by people who have been conditioned into thinking that eating meat will result in their health and happiness. (Side note: A 2012 study by Beezhold and Johnston published in 'Nutrition Journal' shows happiness improves and stress decreases on a vegetarian diet!). Still, you may not be convinced to leave your meat behind. Well, let us examine some of the many health benefits to a vegetarian diet!

The root of this question is about feeling that you are depriving yourself. If you are thinking this way, you need to open yourself up to the possibility of considering this plant-based paradigm shift. We tried to convince you in Chapter Four that you can be nutritionally efficient as a vegetarian, but so what? What do you have to gain? Essentially, everything. Better clarity. Increased productivity. More energy. Better fitness levels Better sex (if you believe the PETA commercials). Basically, a better life. First, let's elaborate on this as the author is obviously biased.

Health Benefits

Anyone can give you anecdotal evidence on what *they* think is great (or not so great) about a vegetarian diet, but my mother taught you to be skeptical. So let us look at what science say about a vegetarian diet.

Luckily for us, in the last decade, there has been an increase in studies highlighting the benefits of a vegetarian diet. Studies in the last five years alone have found that plant-based eating has been linked to decreased instances of heart disease, lower risk of cancers, lower blood pressure and cholesterol, and lower risk of osteoporosis (on plant-based calcium and repair). In addition to this, vegetarians experience fewer instances of kidney disease, rheumatoid arthritis, and lower rates of diabetes.

For now, let's focus on one 2013 study conducted by the University of Oxford. Francesca Crowe, who led the study, found that vegetarians are one-third less likely to be hospitalized or die from heart disease than meat and fish eaters. Previous research has suggested that non-meat eaters have fewer heart problems, but it wasn't clear if other lifestyle differences, such as exercise and smoking habits, also played a part.

Crowe and her colleagues tracked almost 45,000 people living in England and Scotland. The study cohort initially reported on their diet, lifestyle and general health beginning in the 1990s. At the start of the study, about a third said that they ate a vegetarian diet without meat or fish. Over the next 12 years, 1086 subjects were hospitalized for heart disease and 169 died.

After taking into account all extenuating factors, the research team found that vegetarians were 32% less likely to develop heart disease than carnivores. The lower heart risk was likely due to lower cholesterol and blood pressure among vegetarians in the study. "If people want to reduce their risk of heart disease by changing their diet, one way of doing that is to follow a vegetarian diet," Crowe told Reuters Health.

Remember that just because you are running on plants, it shouldn't give way to smoking, drinking and slacking off at the gym. Your average vegetarian, however, tends to be more health-conscious and that could also explain why we live an average of six years longer (vegans 10 years) than our meat-eating counterparts.

There is also evidence that people who already have diseases such as cancer, diabetes, and heart disease see improvements over time when they switch to a balanced vegetarian diet. Meat has known carcinogenic elements that alter our cells, and when you stop eating it, the body has a chance to heal itself with life-affirming foods. This could be the reason why meat-eaters who become vegetarian see health improvements. But who cares about the specifics – just try it and see if it works out for yourself!

Practical Benefits

Speaking of working out, vegetarians can make it look easy, naturally. It is well known that vegetarians tend to be thinner than their meat-eating brethren. Because vegetarians have lower BMIs, they find it easier to lose weight and keep it off, giving them more energy.

I think the best reason to try a vegetarian diet is the effect it may have on your mood. Many types of meat are high in arachidonic acid, a non-essential fatty acid. Some researchers have found a link between diets high in arachidonic acid and mood swings. As you may have guessed by now, vegetarians do not have high amounts of arachidonic acid in their diets. Coupled with the obvious health benefit, it's no wonder that we are typically happier than our meat-eating counterparts!

There are many more benefits to being a vegetarian, both health-related and practical. Decreased risk of disease? Lower cholesterol and blood pressure? Check. More energy? Check. Plus much more. So, if you've been having trouble sticking to your diet because your neighbors keep grilling delicious-smelling steaks, just remember that chances are you are likely to be healthier (and possibly happier) than they are!

CHAPTER SEVEN: ISN'T IT DIFFICULT GOING VEGETARIAN?

Well, that all depends on you, doesn't it? It is never really a question about food. It's about discipline. It's about being informed but not inundated. It's about self-experimenting but not to the extreme. It's about life, growth and an abundance of natural energy. Once you agree with these points, you will have enough leverage to flourish and not fail.

Some people have a hard time cutting meat out of their diets, and would probably do best if they made the transition slowly. A lifetime in our Western society surrounded by the marketing of meat can do that to you. Those who never ate much meat to begin with will have an easier time making the change. With that in mind, let's take a look at the physiological and psychological blocks that might make going vegetarian difficult, and the best ways to avoid them.

Psychological

Maybe you feel that you cannot live without your steaks, hamburgers and bacon. The very thought makes you want to cry. Is the plate half full or half empty?

For some, they won't consider it a full meal without meat. This can be a difficult thing to overcome if you're used to having meat with every meal. The fact that you aren't seeing a slab on your plate can make you believe that you aren't getting all of the nutrients you need or that you aren't full when the meal is finished. Thinking like this can actually be a serious block to getting your

V-plates. However, there are some tricks to move past it.

First, learn to love legumes. Try eating foods like chickpeas, lentils, and beans. They are versatile, protein-rich (which is what most meat-eaters claim they aren't getting enough of) and are filling. The reason meat makes you feel full isn't the protein or even the weight of it; it's the saturated fats that are prevalent in meat. Once you find a good replacement for feeling like you are full, you'll move past this particular block in no time.

Second, some feel that there isn't enough variety in vegetarian meals. I initially thought this as well. But ironically, it's a welcomed paradox. For every cut of meat you give up, there are 1000's of different types of legumes, nuts or grains you've never eaten, let alone heard of. In addition to this, for every type of meat, there are 1000's of fruit and veggies waiting to be trialed that you've never eaten. You're limited by your imagination. There are entire cookbooks full of easy-to-make vegetarian recipes that will leave you full and satisfied. As a free bonus for purchasing this book, you'll find two complimentary books (plus a juice cheat sheet) to download at vegebody.com/amazongifts that will get you started.

Physiological

Do I have to worry about meat withdrawal?

This is not an issue unless you haven't done a good job balancing your new diet. Some people get headaches or feel lethargic after cutting meat from their diets, but if you are careful to make sure that your new vegetarian diet is replacing things like iron and certain vitamins, you will be fine. As well, sometimes there can be withdrawal symptoms from the chemicals in processed meats (yes, just like smoking), but that is a blessing and not a curse.

Will going vegetarian make me gassy?

Gas is actually more a problem of the combination of foods. When initially changing your diet, your body has to find a way to adjust to the digestive demands. This is something that will regulate itself as your body gets used to the higher nutrient intake, particularly fiber.

Am I getting all the nutrients from this diet?

This can be a legitimate problem if you aren't careful about planning your diet. While you make the switch, it can be beneficial to take supplements like iron and vitamin B12, however, consult a good ‚plant-based' doctor or practitioner in your city first.

Just like any lifestyle change, going vegetarian has its difficulties. However, if you're serious about it and proactive in the way you approach your new diet, many of the psychological and physiological effects of going vegetarian are easily mitigated and will become non-existent.

On the flip side, some people feel that vegetarianism helps them stay in tune with their spiritual side. Others feel a sense of relief that they no longer have to hurt innocent animals for their own nourishment. Vegetarianism can also help you learn to be more aware of your surroundings, and especially what you put in your mouth. (For one thing, you would probably start reading the label on food products, and at the same time you'll realize how many junky chemicals are put into processed foods.)

The changes you may experience once you become a vegetarian are subjective, but if you do things right, you will definitely find that a vegetarian diet is so much better for your body and for your fitness goals than a regular diet that includes meat. You just have to try it before you knock it!

Now, just remember that what you feel about leaving animal products behind, will eventually fade once you take the steps toward becoming a vegetarian. You have to approach going vegetarian in the right way so that you don't ,toss your salad in the air' and reach for a burger instead.

CHAPTER EIGHT: HOW CAN AN ELITE ATHLETE BE PLANT-BASED?

Can vegetarians perform as well as their carnivorous counterparts in competition?

Of course, and by the end of this chapter we hope to dispel this myth.

Let's begin by name-dropping from some seriously adrenaline-kicking athletes…

- Joe Namath (legendary quarterback, NFL Hall of Fame 1985)

- Martina Navratilova and Billie Jean King (two of the greatest tennis players of the 20th Century)

- Mac Danzig (US Mixed Martial Arts fighter)

- Bill Pearl (five-time Mr. Universe champion)

- Carl Lewis (10 Olympic track and field medals, nine of them gold)

- Robert Parish (One of the greatest NBA basketball players in history)

- Dave Scott (record for most Iron Man world championship victories ever)

Lizzie Armitstead, an Olympic medal winner in the 87-mile cycling race, recently wrote a book called "Running with the Kenyans". In the book, she mentions that a typical Kenyan athlete's diet is predominately plant-based and meat is usually reserved for special occasions. These athletes live mostly on rice, beans and vegetables. The list of gold medal Kenyan athletes alone is overwhelming.

Many conventional nutritionists are still unconvinced of the benefits of a vegetarian diet for elite sportspeople. While it can mean a diet low in saturated fat, it still requires athletes to be more vigilant about where they get their other nutrients. It is hard work, but as an exercise physiologist, Dr. Darren Morton says, "It's a question that's already been answered because so many athletes have shown that it can be done."

There is a stigma that athletes must stuff their bodies full of protein-packed meats in order to be successful in their sports. Where did that idea come from? Does meat naturally make you into some kind of Herculean human? No, it does not. It is quite the opposite. Let's talk about some of the myths surrounding vegetarians and their supposed inability to be elite athletes.

Can Vegetarians Really Be Athletes?

Vegetarians can, of course, be among the top athletes without having to fill their bodies with foods that will ultimately harm them. What one eats is only part of the equation for top athletes. Animal fats are not magic and do not make a person stronger. Vegetarian diets are typically nutrient-rich live (oxygen-rich) foods, being derived mostly from nature (fruits, vegetables, legumes, nuts, etc.), which replenishes the body, feeds the muscles and cleans out the lymphatic system faster, which makes them stronger. You can, of course, make mistakes with a vegetarian diet and will likely be dealing with the same issues as other elite athletes. As with any high-performance diet, it is imperative to limit processed foods and increase the amount of protein and vegetables you consume. Vegetarians will become strong and increase their endurance by eating foods like nuts, tofu, and beans.

You Can't Create Muscles From Vegetables Alone, Can You?

Well, this is true to some extent, but it is another unfortunate misconception. Vegetarians are not rabbits. There are hundreds of foods in the vegetarian diet besides simple lettuce and carrot sticks. There is no limit to the variety of foods that vegetarians can enjoy. Think of everything from burgers to casseroles. The only difference is that vegetarians are filling their bodies with foods that are healthier, closer to nature and more nutritious, thus adding healthy bulk to their bodies.

Yet, as Olympic cyclist Lizzie Armitstead has shown, vegetarians continue to rise to the very top of their sports. She follows a long line of Olympians who have managed to excel without "eating corpses" as she herself puts it.

As one report said, "It's hard to imagine Rocky Balboa shaping up for a fight on veggie burgers but, hey, he's only a movie character." In real life, US boxers Timothy Bradley and even Mike Tyson have turned vegetarian. More interesting still, Bradley is a self-confessed meat lover, but when it comes to training for an event, he says an all-plant diet with no animal products works best for him.

Scott Jurek, a vegan ultra-runner, recently published his autobiography "Eat & Run", where he explains why he turned vegetarian and then vegan. It wasn't simply for ethics or health, but to run faster. He ran the Minnesota Voyageur 50-mile race three times before he won. The only difference he identified on that third occasion was diet.

"I won the Voyageur on my third try, eating more plants and less meat. I didn't run harder. I was right: I couldn't run harder. But I had learned something important. I could run smarter. I could eat smarter."
Maybe there's something to that: giving more thought to what we eat, considering its provenance and assessing how it makes us feel as runners could lead to changed and improved diets, whether vegetarian or not. Such awareness of what works for our bodies can undoubtedly help us reach the holy grail of peak athletic performance.

Jurek credits his astonishing runs of 160 kilometres on being fuelled by foods like quinoa porridge with almond milk. Interspersed with accounts of brutal races up mountains and across deserts in blistering heat, are recipes for Minnesota winter chilli, apple cinnamon granola, and other vegan dishes for endurance. Jurek is convinced that making the switch from a diet big on barbecues, burgers and fries improved his performance – although he's not sure whether it's because of what he's eating or what he's leaving out, like trans-fats and refined carbohydrates.

"There is no reason that someone who eats a vegan or vegetarian diet can't build just as much muscle as an omnivore," says Matt Ruscigno, MPH, RD. "They can get all of the same amino acids in the right amounts." By using plant-based protein powders in your pre and post lifting snacks, you'll assist your body with natural proteins. It is especially important to mix up your powders, rotating through several types in order to consume a variety of nutrients from different sources.

So, Can Elite Athletes Really be Plant-Based?

There's US basketball player Robert Parish, marathon runner Robert de Castella, tennis player Martina Navratilova, Bill Pearl, who won the 1971 Mr. Universe title as a vegetarian, and track and field Olympian Carl Lewis, who have all said they performed best on a plant-based diet.

"When it comes to high-end performance, a high carbohydrate intake is important for endurance events as well as for power and strength and this is what plants can provide," explains Morton, a senior lecturer in health and exercise science at Avondale College of Further Education in Lake Macquarie. As for the extra protein required for serious bodybuilding or strength, there is an endless choice of plant-based protein powders for protein shakes.

Does A Vegetarian Diet Have Any Added Benefits For Athletic Performance?

There is still minimal research being done on the subject, but according to Morton from the Australian Institute of Sport, he wonders if the extra plant foods might reduce the number of sick days that keep athletes away from training. Although regular moderate exercise is considered an immune system booster, some research suggests that the stress of strenuous training at an elite level can make athletes more susceptible to colds and flu.

"It may be that a vegetarian diet is protective. If you eat a plant-based diet you are getting a lot of extra antioxidants from vegetables and fruit so you're less likely to get sick as often and you can front up for training every day," suggests Morton, who's also a recreational triathlete who has followed a vegan diet (if you don't count chocolate, he says!) for over four years.

If there's a downside to vegetarian eating for athletes, especially vegan diets that skip dairy products and eggs, it's that plant foods tend to be low in kilojoules.

"Athletes who train at a high level need to work at eating a lot of food in order to get enough kilojoules," Morton says. "But for non-athletes that can be an advantage of a vegan diet – you can still eat more food and weigh less."

High-intensity activity requires higher levels of protein, calcium, iron and vitamin B12 (all those things we covered in chapter four), so vegetarian athletes must be creative enough to combine these nutrients at meal time to meet their needs.

I have been a very active vegetarian most of my adult life and am proud of the fact that despite what some people perceive as a restricted diet, I very rarely get sick. In fact, increased health and fitness was initially the sole reason I first became vegetarian. At my peak, I was 108kg with 8% body fat purely on a 100% natural plant-based diet.

CHAPTER NINE: CONCLUSION

At the end of the day, the research presented on plant-based eating should be the catalyst for prompting your own lifestyle change. After all, any issue worth contending will always have well-thought-out viewpoints.

When it comes to your health and fitness, it is simple. By using your common sense, you'll get the results you want quicker. Sticking closer to natural sources, the way nature intended, will always be the healthier option.

Beyond both the documented and anecdotal health advantages, people choose vegetarianism for a number of reasons. And when they do, they will inevitably face questions from others and even themselves regarding whether eating a plant-based diet really is worth it.

I hope this book has provided you with answers or at least has prompted you to ask more of the right questions when going plant-based. The key is to continue the evolution of you. This will happen only with continual learning, self-experimentation and staying the course. A good next step is to check out the research papers, websites, and links in the recommended readings section.

Thanks for taking the time to expand your knowledge ongoing plant-based, and all the best should you choose to go green.

Clay Elston

2016

RECOMMENDED RESOURCES

Nutrition Books & DVD's

The China Study by T. Colin Campbell

The Plant-Powered Diet by Sharon Palmer

Thrive by Brendan Brazier

Eating Animals by Jonathan Safran Foer

Forks Over Knives (DVD)

Vegucated (DVD)

Cowspiracy (DVD)

Earthlings (DVD)

Cookbooks

Thug Kitchen: Eat like you give a f*ck,

Veganomicon by Isa Chandra Moskowitz and Terry Hope Romero

Clean Foods by Terry Walters

Fitness

Fit for Life by Harvey Diamond

Eat and Run by Scott Jurek

Finding Ultra by Rich Roll

Shred Up by Robert Cheeke

Podcasts

No Meat Athlete Podcast (www.nomeathlete.com)
The Rich Roll Podcast (www.richroll.com)
Vegan Body Revolution Show
(www.veganbodyrevolution.com)

Websites

Vege Body (www.vegebody.com)
Happy Cow (www.happycow.net)
No Meat Athlete (www.nomeatathlete.com)
Veg News (www.vegnews.com)
Vegan Bodybuilding and Fitness
(www.veganbodybuilding.com)

Habit Software

Trello (www.trello.com)
StickK (www.stickk.com)
Evernote (www.evernote.com)
7 Weeks – Habit and Goal Tracker (Android App)
Habit Bull (Android App)
Momentum (Apple App)

DON'T FORGET YOUR COMPLIMENTARY BONUSES!

To make sure you get the most value out of a book about going vegetarian, here are three exclusive resources that will help you on your vegetarian journey.

1. 1000 Vegetarian Recipes

We compiled 1000 delicious recipes for all occasions and it is yours for purchasing this book on Amazon. You'll never need another recipe book again!

2. Juice Cheat Sheet

This is a one page print off with 24 of my favourite juices. Print it off and stick it in your kitchen. It's the perfect "cheat sheet" when you need to get your ‚juices' flowing!

3. All Time Favourites

This is a beautifully designed curated collection of our favourite recipes.

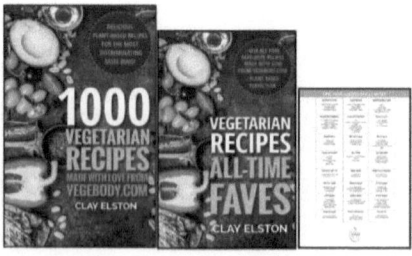

You can download these resources here:
www.vegebody.com/amazongifts

THANKS FOR READING. NOW, WHAT?

Dear Reader,

Before you go, sincere thanks for reading this book. I hope you received value from it as much as I did in writing it.

If you enjoyed this book, I would love an honest review since the success of this book relies largely on Amazon reviews.

I would love to hear valuable feedback and helpful comments as this will help with future updates. Feel free to email me through www.vegebody.com.

Lastly, no animals were harmed in the creation of any of my books.

With gratitude,
Clay Elston